KU-490-291

GO FACTS **HEALTHY BODIES**

Health

Susan Mansfield

9030 00000 9427 3

Health

© 2007 Blake Publishing
Additional material © A & C Black Publishers Ltd 2009

First published in Australia by Blake Education Pty Ltd.

This edition published in the United Kingdom in 2009 by
A & C Black Publishers Ltd, 36 Soho Square, London, W1D 3QY.
www.acblack.com

Published by permission of Blake Publishing Pty Ltd, Leichhardt NSW, Australia.

All rights reserved. No part of this publication may be reproduced in any form or by
any means – graphic, electronic or mechanical, including photocopying, recording,
taping or information storage and retrieval systems – without the prior written
permission of the publishers.

Hardback edition
ISBN 978-1-4081-1225-0

Paperback edition
ISBN 978-1-4081-1224-3

A CIP record for this book is available from the British Library.

Written by Susan Mansfield
Publisher: Katy Pike
Editor: Mark Stafford
Design and layout by The Modern Art Production Group.

Photo credits: p9–Diagram and recommendations based on CSIRO research and the
12345+ Food and Nutrition Plan, produced by M. Jackson, Anti-Cancer Foundation,
South Australia, in turn based on Baghurst KI, Hertzler AA, Record SJ, Spur C. 1992.
The development of a simple dietary assessment and education tool... Journal of
Nutritional Education 24: 165–172. p27–Getty Images

Printed in China by WKT Company Ltd.

This book is produced using paper that is made from wood grown in managed
sustainable forests. It is natural, renewable and recyclable. The logging and
manufacturing processes conform to the environmental regulations of the country
of origin.

LONDON BOROUGH OF WANDSWORTH	
9030 00000 9427 3	
Askews	29-Apr-2010
C613 MANS	£4.99
	WWX0006293/0058

What is Health?

Health is a person's physical, mental and spiritual wellbeing.

A healthy body

Physical health is more than not being ill. It means being fit enough to do all the things a person needs to do.

Regular physical activity is the best way to get fit and healthy. It reduces stress and heart disease, strengthens bones, and helps to maintain a healthy body weight. Diet also affects physical health.

A healthy mind

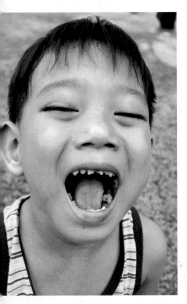

Mental health is the **mind's** health. It includes a person's feelings, and how they affect life.

Mental health involves positive experiences, like happiness and peace, as well as negative experiences, like stress and depression.

Just as there are many levels of physical health, there are many levels of mental health. Signs of good mental health include feeling **competent**, being able to handle normal levels of stress, and having a positive outlook on life.

Spiritual wellbeing

Spirituality means different things to different people, but it usually includes belief in something greater than oneself. This gives life a sense of meaning.

Spirituality can take many forms. It may include religion, nature, or a set of values to live by.

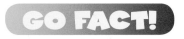

OLDEST
Frenchwoman Jeanne Calment was 122 years 164 days when she died in 1997.

Eating many different foods helps maintain a healthy, interesting diet.

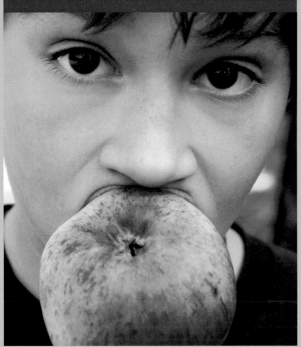

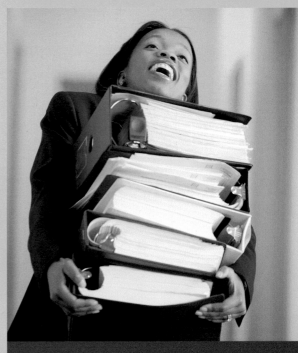

The number one reason for not exercising: 'I don't have enough time'.

Walking for 30 minutes every day improves health.

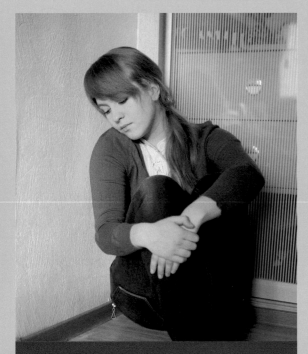

Up to a quarter of young people experience depression by the age of 18.

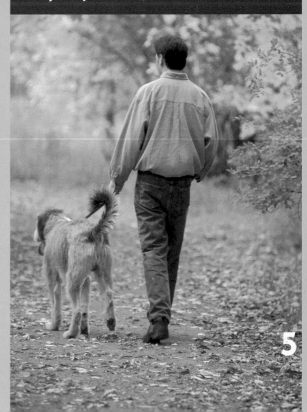

What Does the Body Need?

The body needs food for energy and growth, and sleep for rest and repair.

Nutrients

Nutrients are substances that help the body live and grow. The six types of nutrients are:

- carbohydrates – to supply energy
- fats – to supply energy and build structures in the body
- proteins – to supply energy and build structures, and they are required for body processes, eg digestion
- vitamins – required for body processes, eg vitamin A for vision
- minerals – required for body processes, eg sodium for nerves and muscles
- water – needed by every cell in the body.

Energy to burn

Food is converted to energy in a process called **metabolism**. The most common source of energy is carbohydrate. Foods rich in carbohydrates include bread, rice and potatoes. If it is resting, the body can supply all its energy needs for about 12 hours from stored carbohydrates.

A good night's sleep

Sleep is important for good brain development. It is essential for normal speech, memory and thinking. For example, staying awake for 17 hours straight makes a person behave as though they are at the top of the legal blood alcohol level.

People aged 10–12 need about nine hours of sleep every night.

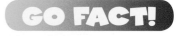

GO FACT!

LONGEST

The record for the longest period without sleep is 11 days, but sleep deprivation is very dangerous.

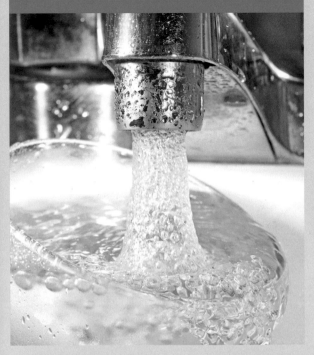

Some tap water in the UK contains fluoride, a chemical which strengthens teeth.

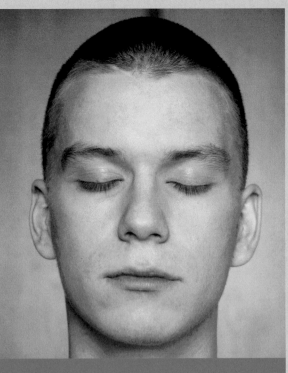

People typically spend more than two hours each night dreaming.

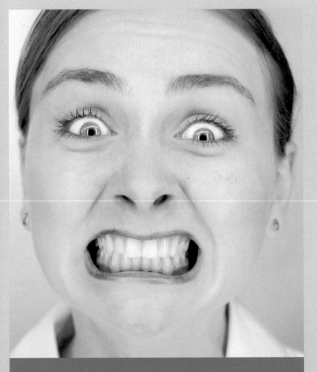

Most minerals are stored in the bones and teeth.

Exercise every day – a tired body is more likely to sleep well.

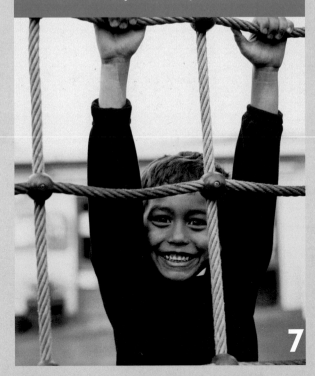

Food Groups

A balanced diet means eating the right amounts from each of the five food groups.

Meat and meat alternatives

This group provides protein and vitamin B12, and the minerals iron and zinc. The best choice from this group is **lean**, red meat. Poultry, fish, eggs and pulses (eg beans, lentils) do not provide as much iron and zinc as red meat. Meat should be trimmed of fat and cooked without using extra fat.

Milk and milk products

Milk, yoghurt and cheese provide protein, fat, salt, zinc and calcium. They are important for strong bones and teeth. Low-fat products are the best choices.

Fruit

Fruit contains **fibre**, natural sugars, and important vitamins and minerals. The skin on fruit is a good source of fibre. Fruit juice does not usually provide as much fibre as whole fruit. Fruit loses much of its vitamin C when it is dried.

Vegetables

The dark green, leafy vegetables, such as spinach, contain chemicals that fight some cancers. The orange-yellow vegetables, such as carrots, provide vitamin A. Starchy vegetables, such as potatoes, are a good source of carbohydrate.

Breads and cereals

Most breads and cereals provide fibre, protein, vitamins and minerals – **wholegrain** products (muesli, oats and wholegrain breads) provide most.

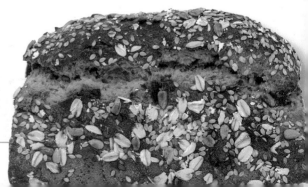

A balanced diet can be described using a food pyramid.

Extras

If you are active and not overweight, you could have one or two of these each day.

Meat and meat alternatives

1 serving per day

(teenagers need one extra meat serving each day)

Examples of one serving: 2 small lamb chops, 2 small eggs, 100 g almonds.

Milk and milk products

2 servings per day

(teenagers need one extra milk serving each day)

Examples of one serving: 1 large glass milk, 40 g cheese, 200 g yoghurt.

Fruit

3 servings per day

Examples of one serving: 1 apple or banana, 10 strawberries, 20 grapes.

Vegetables

4 servings per day

Examples of one serving: 1 potato, $\frac{1}{3}$ carrot, 80 g peas.

Breads and cereals

5 servings per day

(teenagers need 9–12 servings each day)

Examples of one serving: 1 slice bread, 56g cooked pasta, 80 g muesli.

Choose What You Eat

Plan what to eat to maintain good health and a healthy weight.

The energy that you put into your body should balance the energy that your body uses. If you eat too much food, it is stored as fat; too little leaves you tired and weak.

The amount of energy in food is measured in calories (kcal). You'll need paper, a pen and calculator for this procedure.

What to do:

1 Choose the amount of energy you use in a typical day.

	10 – 11 year old girl	10 – 11 year old boy
average level of activity	2 020 – 2 140 kcal per day	2 500 – 2620 kcal per day
very active	2 260 – 2475 kcal per day	2 760 – 3045 kcal per day

2 Plan your meals for a day, including snacks and drinks, from the options on the opposite page. Make sure to choose meals from the five food groups.

3 Add the energy content for the meals you choose. Add or remove items until you reach your energy target.

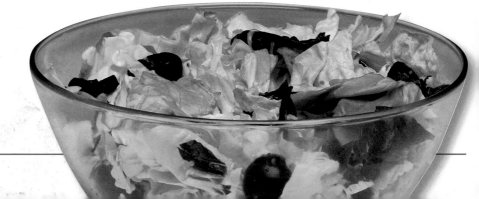

breakfast	energy content (calories)
fruit salad and yoghurt	263
porridge and milk	210
2 wheat biscuits and milk	167
1 piece toast and peanut butter	130
1 piece toast and jam	86

lunch	energy content (calories)
salad roll	289
2 pieces grilled cheese on toast	279
chicken and tomato roll	252
tuna and salad sandwich	187
vegetable soup	102

dinner	energy content (calories)
roast lamb and vegetables	556
beef and vegetable stir-fry	524
baked fish and vegetables	374
chicken and vegetable pasta	315
chicken salad	262

dessert	energy content (calories)
chocolate cake	345
1 mango	122
3 scoops ice-cream	85
1 kiwifruit	43
80 g strawberries	13

snacks	energy content (calories)
fruit muffin	157
banana	107
1 small can baked beans	77
apple	74
80 g homemade popcorn	42

drinks	energy content (calories)
1 glass chocolate milk	141
1 glass milk	121
1 glass orange juice	86
water	0

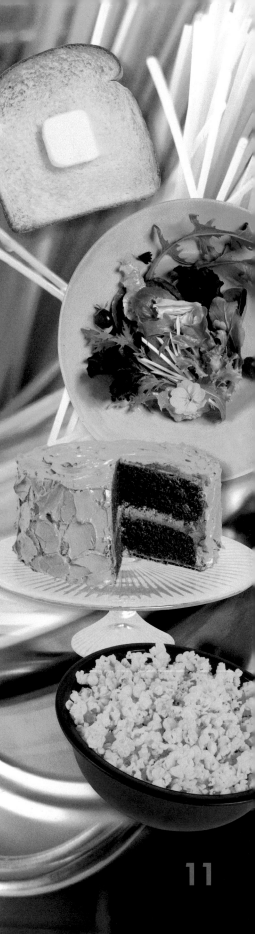

Fast Food

Fast food is inexpensive, and quick to prepare and serve. But it may not be a healthy meal.

Fast food often contains high levels of fat, salt or sugar. It can be low in fibre, vitamins and minerals. It is popular with suppliers because it is cheap to make, lasts a long time and may not need refrigeration.

Some people believe that fast food is harmless when eaten as part of a balanced diet. So-called healthy foods do not always lead to good health. Many snack food bars are sold as health foods, although they are high in sugar and fat.

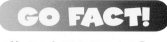

GO FACT!

DID YOU KNOW?

A fast-food strawberry milkshake may contain more than 50 artificial ingredients. A healthier milkshake would contain just strawberries and milk!

Many breakfast cereals are marketed as healthy although they have high levels of sugar.

Generally, replacing healthy meals with fast food too often can lead to vitamin and mineral shortages, heart disease and **obesity**.

Less advertising

People choose food based on what they like, whether it is healthy, and how much time they have to eat.

Advertising also influences food choices. In the UK, all advertising for junk food (food containing high levels of fat, salt and sugar) have been banned from being shown around or during children's TV programmes. This is because of rising levels of childhood obesity.

Many foods contain additives, natural or artificial, which are added to foods for different reasons.

reason	example, including code number
improve taste or appearance	beeswax – glazing agent (901) makes apples shiny
improve quality or stability	sorbitol – humectant (420) helps dried fruit stay moist and soft
preserve food	sulphur dioxide – preservative (220) in sausages stops growth of bacteria that cause food poisoning

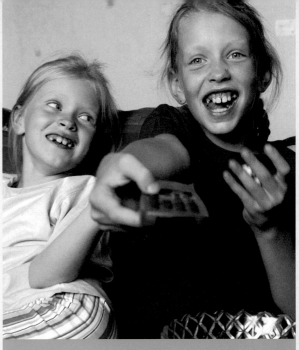

Adverts for food and drink high in fat, salt and sugar have been banned from children's TV in the UK since 2009.

Many fast food meals come in different sizes. Larger meals contain a lot more calories for little extra cost. This causes many people to overeat.

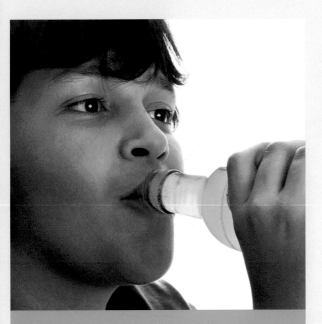

Since the millennium, the number of fizzy drinks British children aged 10-12 consume per year has almost halved – from 30 per cent to 17 per cent.

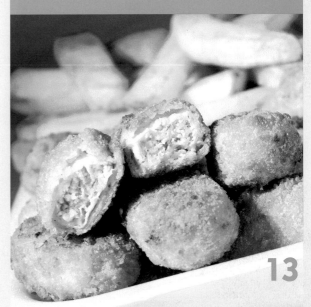

13

Your Body

Your body image is how you feel about your physical appearance.

People naturally focus on what their bodies look like as they grow. There are a lot of influences on body image – friends, family, television, magazines – but many are unrealistic.

For example, the average British woman's dress size is 14. Many fashion designers and magazine editors use tall, thin models, who wear size 10 or smaller. If all models are very thin, it can make girls and women feel that they are the wrong weight and shape.

GO FACT!
DID YOU KNOW?

A man's desire for more muscles may relate to the action figures he liked as a boy.

A distorted image

A negative body image can lead to anxiety and low **self-esteem**. In severe cases, focusing on weight and food can lead to eating disorders. People with **anorexia nervosa** look in the mirror and see themselves as fat, even though they are very underweight. **Binge** eaters consume large amounts of food at one time, even when they are not hungry. These disorders are problems for males and females.

It's your body

The body's **genes** determine its height and body shape, just as they determine skin colour. People are happier when they concentrate on making healthy choices, such as eating well and exercising regularly.

Every image of a model or actress in a magazine has been adjusted using computers to remove bulges, spots and marks.

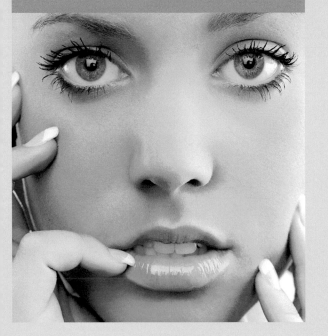

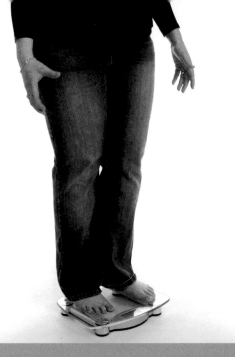

Britons spend millions every year on weight loss programs that have little effect on their weight.

About half of the people with binge eating disorders are male.

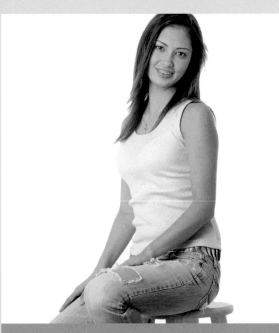

It is normal for women to carry fat on their hips and thighs. It is vital for healthy bones, skin, eyes, hair and teeth.

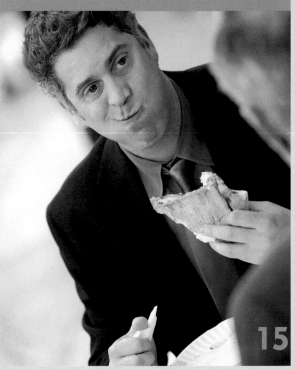

Mental Health

Anxiety, depression, worry and fear are part of life. If they persist or become severe, you should seek help.

Anxiety

During an anxiety or panic attack, a person feels nervous, sweaty and dizzy. The heart races wildly, and it can be hard to breathe. The feeling is very scary and overwhelming.

A treatment for anxiety involves making a chart of the time,

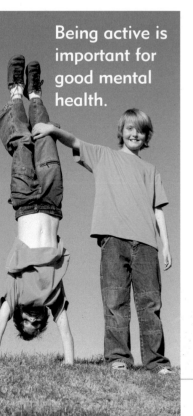

Being active is important for good mental health.

place, breathing rate and activity of the person. Completing this chart four times each day for several weeks helps to identify the situations that trigger anxiety.

Depression

Depression is a serious illness, not a reaction to life. While we all feel sad from time to time, people with depression are intensely sad, for long periods and often without reason.

Depression can be as damaging to a person's life as physical illness and injury.

One in five Britons experience depression at some stage of their lives. Depression may get worse if it is untreated. There are many health services available that provide information, treatment and support. With help, it is possible to recover from depression and enjoy everything life has to offer.

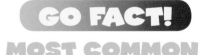

GO FACT!

MOST COMMON

Depression is the most common mental illness experienced by children and teenagers.

Can't stop worrying about something? Try these steps to solve the problem.

1. Write down exactly what you believe the main problem is.
2. Write down all possible solutions, even bad ones.
3. Think about each solution.
4. Choose the most practical solution.
5. Plan how you will carry out that solution.
6. Do it!

If this didn't solve the problem, you may see the problem differently now. If so, write down the problem as you now understand it and repeat the six steps.

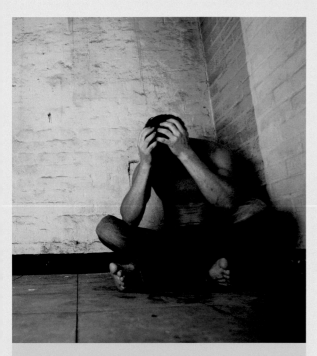

In some countries, people with mental illnesses are treated as criminals.

People who are homeless are more likely to have poor mental health than the general population.

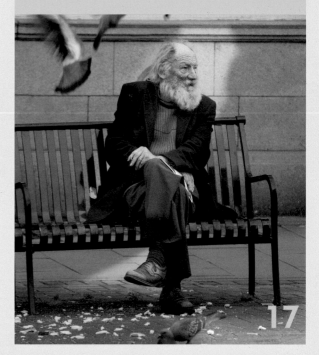

17

Healthy Relationships

All relationships need communication and cooperation to be successful.

Some relationships are closer than others. Some relationships we choose, such as friends, while others are decided for us, such as family and teachers.

Relationships shape how you feel about yourself. Being aware of the way relationships affect you can help you make the right choices in life.

A relationship is healthy when you:

- are accepted for who you are
- can laugh or cry with each other
- listen and understand each other
- feel comfortable, safe and supported.

Bullying

Bullying is another term for being picked on or pushed around. It includes spreading nasty rumours and cyber bullying, which involves sending threatening emails and text messages.

Bullying isn't limited by age or gender. It is found in every school and nursery.

Victims of bullying often feel alone, sad, angry and scared. Bullies often have low self-esteem or have been victims of violence themselves. Bullying is their way of dealing with their own problems.

If you are being bullied it is not your fault and there is nothing wrong with you. Don't be afraid to let a parent or teacher know about it immediately.

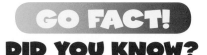

GO FACT!
DID YOU KNOW?

More than two-thirds of children say they are very satisfied with their relationship with their parents.

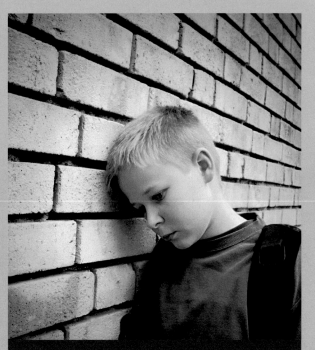

Since 1972, the number of weddings taking place in the UK has fallen dramatically.

One in four British children has parents who live separately.

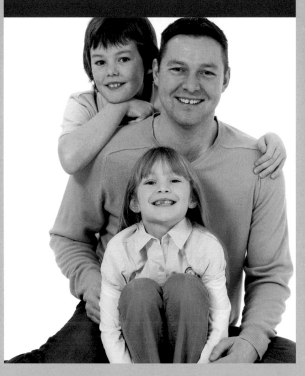

Cyber bullying is the fastest growing form of bullying among school children.

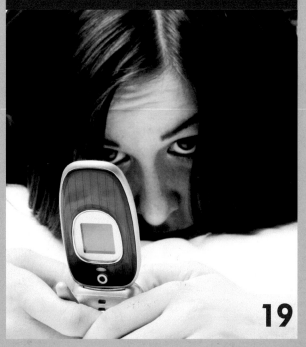

Letting someone get bullied without doing anything about it, makes it look like you agree with it.

Healthy Skin

Skin is the human body's biggest organ. It protects our internal organs, helps to keep our bodies at a healthy temperature and provides our sense of touch.

The body has two main layers of skin. The thin, outer layer is called the epidermis. The cells on its surface are dead and flake off about every two weeks. New skin cells continually rise through the epidermis to replace the dead ones. Beneath the epidermis is the thicker dermis. It contains sweat and sebaceous glands, nerves, hair **follicles** and blood vessels.

Skin changes

Sebaceous glands produce sebum, an oily substance that helps to keep hairs and skin soft and waterproof. As the body enters **puberty** and begins to release **hormones**, it may produce too much sebum. This can block hair follicles and cause spots or **acne**.

Sun and skin

The body needs sunlight to remain healthy, but too much can be dangerous. Sunburn can permanently damage the skin and increases the chances of skin cancer. The only cure for sunburn is slow healing. It can be easily avoided by using sunscreen, wearing protective clothing (especially a hat) and staying out of the sun in the middle of the day.

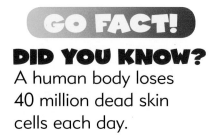

GO FACT!

DID YOU KNOW?
A human body loses 40 million dead skin cells each day.

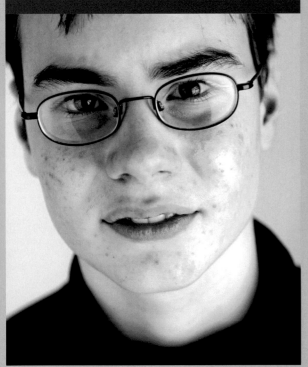

Stress can trigger an outbreak of spots.

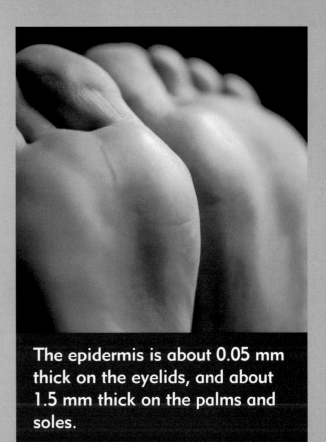

The epidermis is about 0.05 mm thick on the eyelids, and about 1.5 mm thick on the palms and soles.

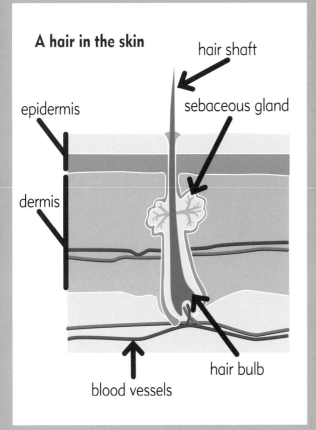

A hair in the skin

hair shaft

sebaceous gland

epidermis

dermis

hair bulb

blood vessels

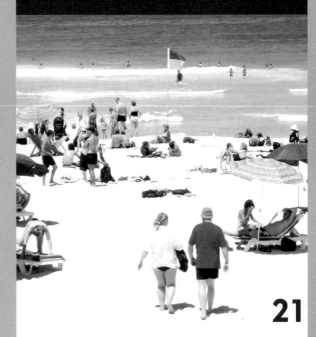

Australia and New Zealand have the highest rates of melanoma (skin cancers) in the world.

21

Healthy Teeth

Healthy, strong teeth are important for chewing food and speaking clearly.

Dental problems

Within 20 minutes of eating, plaque begins to build up on teeth. Plaque is a sticky film of bacteria and food that causes tooth decay. It attacks tooth enamel, which is the outer layer of a tooth, and creates holes (cavities). Sugary foods and drinks increase the risk of cavities. A 375 millilitre can of soft drink contains about 10 teaspoons of sugar.

Plaque also causes bad breath and gum disease. Gum disease makes gums red and swollen, and if untreated may cause teeth to die and fall out. It has also been linked to heart disease and diabetes.

Care of teeth

Healthy teeth are clean and have few cavities. Healthy gums are pink and firm. Brushing with a soft toothbrush at least twice each day is the main way to keep teeth and gums healthy. The tongue should also be brushed to remove bacteria that cause bad breath.

Flossing each day removes trapped food. Regular cleaning by a dentist removes plaque that may develop even with careful brushing and flossing.

Calcium in milk is vital for healthy teeth.

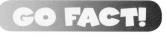

GO FACT!

HARDEST

Tooth enamel is the hardest material in the body – even harder than bone.

The dentist's mirror shows tooth decay behind the front teeth (incisors).

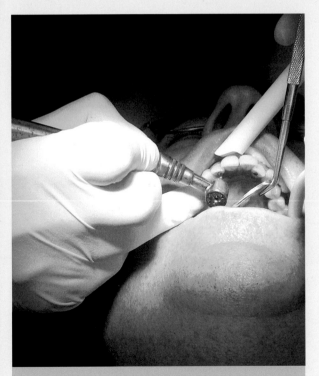

A dentist uses a drill to remove tooth decay.

The first teeth are not permanent – they fall out and are replaced by new teeth from about age six onwards.

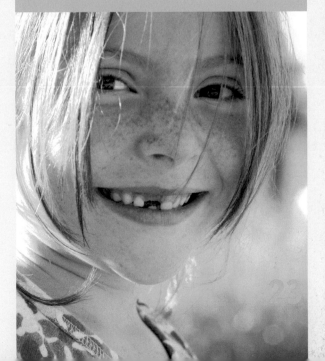

Drugs

A drug is a chemical that changes the way the body works and feels.

Drugs come from many sources. Some are from plant or animal extracts, some from live bacteria. Others are made in laboratories.

Some drugs are helpful – others are harmful.

Medicinal drugs

Medicinal drugs are used to help the body become healthy when things go wrong. If you have a bacterial infection that your body is finding hard to fight, you may be given antibiotics. Antibiotics are drugs that help eliminate infections. Helpful drugs are prescribed by a doctor or are available from a trained pharmacist.

Recreational drugs

Recreational drugs also change the way your body is working, but not in a good way. Using recreational drugs can be harmful. Overuse can lead to dependency and drug addiction. Breaking an addiction causes a lot of physical and mental pain.

Not all users of recreational drugs become addicts, but all recreational drugs are harmful to good health if overused. Many of these drugs, such as ecstasy, heroin and marijuana are also illegal.

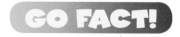

GO FACT!
MOST COMMON

Alcohol is the most widely used drug in Britain.

There is no cure for a hangover – cold showers, exercise, coffee, food, fresh air and vomiting will not take away the pain.

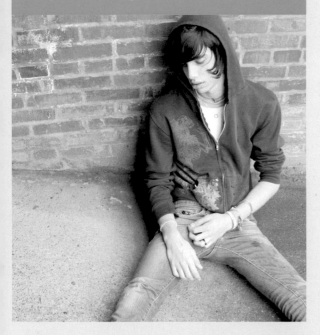

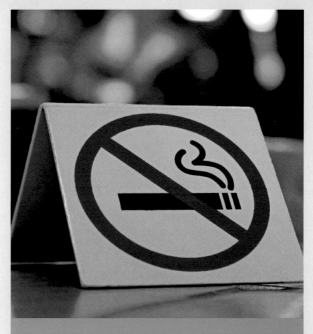

There are more than 4 000 chemicals in tobacco smoke. Many are poisonous and at least 43 cause cancer.

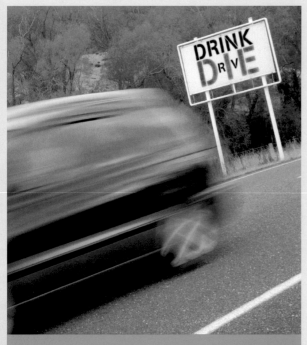

Alcohol causes more than a quarter of all deaths of 15 – 29 year-olds in developed countries.

There are no controls on what is in an illegal drug – it can contain anything. This increases the chances of overdosing and poisoning.

Choosing Health

Living a healthy life is usually a choice. The decisions we make every day affect our health, now and in the future.

Making healthy choices isn't always easy, but it's your life – look after it!

Positive messages

Governments and community groups run **campaigns** to promote good health.

For example, pictures of the effects of smoking, including lung cancer and heart disease have been added to text warnings on cigarette packets. This campaign makes people think more about the risks of smoking, and then try to quit the habit.

Health campaigns show that there are always alternatives to unhealthy decisions. Their message is to respect yourself because you are worth it.

Many voices

Parents, friends, religion, culture, product labels and advertising all have something to say about what is healthy and what isn't.

The alcohol industry spends more than £100 million each year advertising its products. Children aged 13 – 17 years may be exposed to more alcohol advertising on television than people old enough to legally buy alcohol.

Young people are a target for alcohol advertising because they are future adult buyers.

No matter what the product, a smart consumer thinks about the message and asks: Is it good for my health?

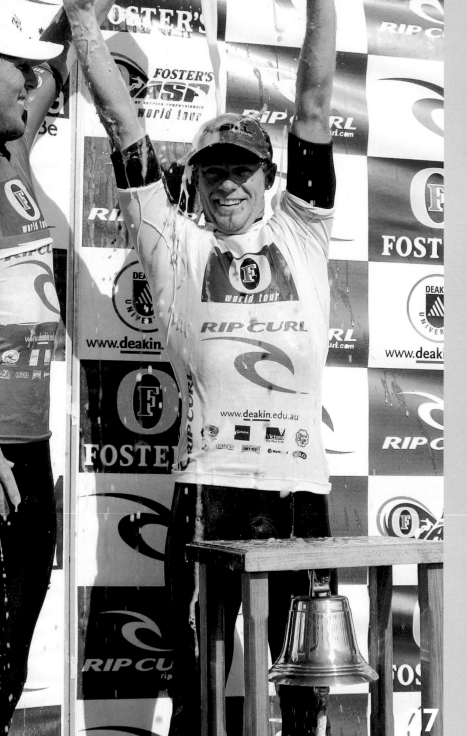

Alcohol companies sponsor sports events. Sponsorship can lead a person to associate a product with youth, health, success and enjoyment.

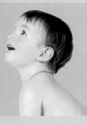

Health Through Life

Before birth

Starting as a single cell, the body grows 5 million times bigger until birth nine months later. The body grows faster at this time than at any other stage in life.

Birth – 12 months

The heart rate of a newborn baby is a 120 beats per minute, almost twice as fast as an adult. Babies cry when they are hungry, lonely or in pain. Drinking only milk at first, they eat solid food from about six months. A baby's weight triples during this period.

1 – 2 years

Infants need more energy for their weight than adults. As physical ability develops, toddlers learn to draw, play with blocks and feed themselves. They begin to feel jealousy, fear and impatience. A two year-old is about half the height he or she will be as an adult.

16 – 19 years

Both genders continue to grow until about 18. The brain is still forming its ability to assess risky behaviour. Peer-group influences are strong. School exams cause stress. Some teenagers enter the workforce.

20s and 30s

A time of social change – work, travel, possibly relationships and children. **Fertility** is at its peak in the early twenties and declines in the late thirties. People establish healthy eating and exercise habits to carry into later life.

40s and 50s

Some people put on weight as metabolism slows. Hair turns grey. Many men lose their hair. Women cease having children. People seek satisfaction through family, work and giving to society.

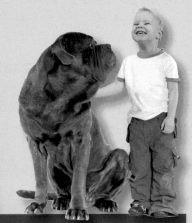

3 – 5 years

Children learn to share and make friends. Nursery age children begin to write and dress themselves. They can balance on one foot and speak in long, grammatically correct sentences. They start their own activities, rather than copying others.

6 – 10 years

Children develop a sense of their worth. They learn to read and write, and can understand concepts such as fantasy and reality. Permanent teeth replace baby teeth.

11 – 15 years

Puberty triggers a growth spurt. (Girls usually begin puberty before boys.) Body shape changes, and sexual organs mature. Puberty also changes thinking and behaviour. Teenagers form their own ideas, morals and values, and rely less on parents for knowledge about life.

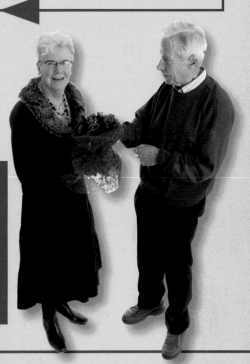

60s and 70s

People eat less – they lose weight and physical strength. Skin develops deeper wrinkles. Sight, hearing and memory may worsen. Bones become weaker and thinner. Most people retire from work. They review their lives, deal with loss and prepare for their last years.

80s and beyond

Mobility is often limited. After 85 years, about half of all people will be affected by some form of **dementia**. Remaining active can prolong good health for many years.

A balanced diet means using the same amount of energy that you eat. Regularly eating more calories than your body needs leads to weight gain.

What's in a fast food burger, large French fries and 600 millilitres of soft drink?

protein	30 grams
fat	49.8 grams
carbohydrates	85.8 grams
sugars	69.7 grams
total energy	1 192 calories

What could you do to use this amount of energy?

	amount of exercise needed by someone weighing about 40 kilograms to use 1 192 calories
row in a race	1 hour 52 minutes
run	4 hours 15 minutes
walk rapidly	8 hours 47 minutes
stand	59 hours 24 minutes
watch television	73 hours 22 minutes

This is an approximate guide – the number of calories used per day depends on many things, including age, weight and level of activity.

Glossary

acne (noun) a skin disease caused by inflamed oil glands, in which small red spots appear on the face and neck

anorexia nervosa (noun) a serious illness in which a person does not eat, or eats too little, because they fear becoming overweight

binge (noun) when something is done in an extreme way, especially eating, drinking or spending money

campaign (noun) a planned group of activities intended to achieve an aim

competent (adjective) able to do something well

dementia (noun) a condition that affects predominantly older people, causing gradual worsening of the memory and other mental abilities

drug dependent (adjective) describes someone who continues to use a drug despite not getting the same effect from it (so they use more) and despite its ill effects

fertility (noun) the ability to produce offspring

fibre (noun) a substance in foods, such as fruit and vegetables, which travels through the body as waste and helps digestion

fit (verb) to become suddenly ill, unconscious and unable to control movements; also (adjective) healthy and strong, especially because of exercise

follicle (noun) a small hole in the skin, especially one that a hair grows from

genes (noun) the specific chemical patterns in a cell that are received from parents and control the development of particular characteristics in an animal or plant

hormone (noun) a chemical made in the body that influences development, growth, sex, etc. and is carried around the body in the blood

lean (adjective) describes meat that has little fat

metabolism (noun) all the chemical changes in the body considered together, especially those that cause food to be used for energy and growth

mind (noun) the part of a person that enables them to think, feel emotions and be aware of things

obesity (noun) being extremely overweight

puberty (noun) when the reproductive organs mature; it is usually ages 10 – 14 for girls and 13 – 16 for boys, although everyone is different

self-esteem (noun) belief and confidence in your ability and value

spirituality (noun) the quality of being concerned with deep feelings and beliefs, rather than with the physical parts of life

unconsciousness (noun) the state of having lost awareness

wellbeing (noun) the state of feeling healthy and happy

wholegrain (adjective) describes foods containing whole grains, not just the inside of the grains

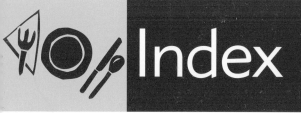

Index

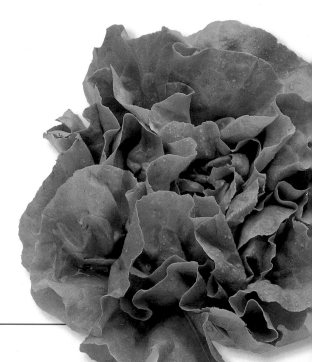